The Unconventional

&
Unorthodox

Things to live by.

By

Stan Dixon

Edited by
James "Sunny" Peel

"On the store counter where it says give a penny take a penny, I say let's up it to a quarter, Times are hard."

~Stan D.

35 AND OVER PLEASE READ

I am forty three years of age and still in pretty good shape. I always been told we lose about a pound of muscle a year after age 35. I'm not in the gym at the present time but I still take glutamine to stop muscle wasting as well as other amino acid and supplements. I only can describe it this way. My muscles are standing still in time while I go on with my day to day life. Not to be a buzz kill but, I firmly believe that age 35 is the perfect time to taper off. Whatever you've consumed (food, alcohol etc.) between the ages of 18 and 34 should be halved starting at age 35.

I try to make sure to keep my body in an alkaline state by staying away from acidic foods. There are PH strips to test alkalinity. If you get acid indigestion it is a good chance that you are acidic. You will want to correct that immediately or it can negatively impact your digestive system and your other ten body systems as well. Start eating salads that consist of kale, onions and carrots. A balanced salad will give nutrient co-factors that also could help with enzyme activity. Tomatoes are acidic so try to omit them for a little while or until you get to a good alkaline base. Some prescriptions could wipe out your enzymes which the body desperately needs to keep a reservoir of. Cancer usually cannot flourish in an alkaline environment.☺ Always consult a Physician before trying anything new.

ARTHUR DOES NOT LIVE HERE ANYMORE

Each day I ask my father how is he feeling and each day he tells me what I already know. That his arthritis is in full swing. Some days are worse than others, particularly the morning after a night at the bar (beer and alcohol may have a direct affect with his uric acid accumulation). Sometimes he is in so much pain. He forgets to take his pills for uric acid, and even when he does sometimes the pills do not work for him. I always try to instill in my father to maximize his medication by drinking plenty of water and cutting back on the saturated fat and yeast products. I'm proud to say my dad is cutting a lot of sugar out of his diet and increasing his water intake, and is joining my gym. We are well on the way to saying "Arthritis does not live here anymore!"

Mere suggestions:

1. CAYENNE PEPPER (pill form)
2. CHERRY JUICE EXTRACT (NO SUGAR)
3. TURMERIC CAPSULES
4. RAW APPLE CIDER VINEGAR
   WITH THE MOTHER INTACT

C F U

CFU is the acronym for colony forming units. They are probiotics (friendly bacteria for a healthy immune system) formulated to set up house in your gut. All probiotics are not created equal. The national commercials do not disclose this in their ads. You have some that are formulated just a tad bit superior to do their job proficiently. Some probiotics are entry coated (protected) to bypass stomach acids ergo acids can kill your probiotics before they get to their targeted destination which is in your gut. Anyone that's on antibiotics, going thru or just getting over a chronic illness may benefit from CFU- So look for CFU on the back label.

Also if your one who gravitates towards the Refrigerated probiotics, just to let you know some of those products come to stores in regular trucks without temperature control. If you're a fanatic about wanting properly shipped refrigerated probiotics check with the vendor of your product and inquire how it is transported.

I learned an interesting thing from old schooler, Robert Gray. Author of "THE COLON HEALTH HANDBOOK" He says that you need to feed your probiotics, ergo they are alive and you want them to flourish to keep you happy. Who would have thought to feed probiotics? The three treats for lacto bacteria growth are onions, cabbage and Jerusalem artichokes. Robert Gray states "One medium to large size onion must be eaten daily to obtain good effect, and it does not matter whether the onion is cooked or raw". TALK TO A KNOWLEDGBLE PHYSICIAN BEFORE USING ANY NEW SUPPLEMENTS.

CHANGE LIKE THE SEASON

At the beginning or in the middle of any season you should detox and receive a massage, ergo the two work in synergy. Prior to writing this piece, I received a massage from a friend and I returned the favor by giving him one as well. He's a massage therapist but he has not had a massage in a year and a half. We know that when people who rarely get massages and finally do so, may experience a detoxifying process. The detox process may create minor flu like symptoms. The reason for starting a detox process at the end of a season is to free yourself of the season's foods and toxins. I suggest starting at the beginning of your vacation or on a Thursday or Friday at the latest, so that you be on track for Mondays hectic work day. Start off with a three day detox or any detox three days before going back to work. You may become lethargic from both the massage and detox and you may ask yourself why you would need to receive a massage if you are taking a detox. Toxins may be harvesting in your muscle fibers that needs to be coached out by a great massage! Always ask your doctor for guidance.

"HIV IS NOT PART OF YOUR
ORIGINAL DNA... SO IT DOES NOT
DEFINE YOU!"

~STAN D.

SAVED BY THE GARLIC

If you feel as if you're catching a cold or that something you ate did not agree with you, it's a foreign invader trying to pillage your village. People try to psyche themselves by drinking some tea and thinking a good night's rest will relieve them of the inevitable. If I consume something that does not agree with me or feel as though a cold is coming on I try to prohibit the replication of the bad bacteria by taking a tip of a tea spoon of garlic powder (not garlic salt) and plenty of water as my first defense against the invaders almost instantly I feel much better.   People often forget that orally they actually promote bad bacteria. Garlic helps kill bacteria in the mouth via the throat, via the rest of your body. Fungus and bad bacteria will grow until it is stopped. Garlic seems to be amazing at helping with inhibiting the procreation of bad bacteria. I use garlic cloves for maintenance, when I feel the onset of a compromised wellbeing I take a quarter teaspoon of garlic powder with meals or until I feel better. If your stomach is sensitive to garlic try to eat and take flax seed or a low to no saturated fat oil with it. Maybe a glass of milk can help with sensitivity to garlic. Remember add a probiotic and always consult with a knowledgeable   physician   before   trying   new supplements.

<u>SAY CHEESE</u>☺

Once upon a time a beautiful lady came into the health food store that I managed she had an awesome smile that "blew me away". She was a little blue. She was out of her brand of tooth paste, Correction toothpowder. The store was also out of the product, but after several weeks it was stocked again. I tried the product myself and I've been hooked ever since. The product is called ECO DENT! I <u>LOVE</u>, <u>LOVE</u>, <u>LOVE</u> IT! The powder hardens my teeth and neutralizes mouth acids. I do brush my teeth with toothpaste in-between uses of ECO DENT for the flouride.

A couple of years ago a friend referred me to his dentist. The dentist made my day. He was excited to find that I did not have not one single cavity. He asked if I whitened my teeth, and I told him "no". He then asked what was I brushing my teeth with and if I could write it down the name for him. WOW!

Second Hand Kiss

May it be second hand smoke or kissing a smoker after they took their much needed drag, you the nonsmoker are ingesting their added bacteria that comes with smoking. Each of us carry bacteria in our periodontal region but some bacteria thrive in heinous anaerobic settings and a smoker's mouth is a prime example. You may notice yourself getting sick more often or wounds healing at a slower rate, or even your beauty products are not working as well. It is possible that being in close proximally with the smoker and with intimate kisses on a regular basis could be the culprit. You should check yourself if you continuously get a smokers cough and you do not smoke. Pollutants particularly cigarette smoke destroys your vitamin C.

I had a friend whose gums would not heal and his dentist suggested it may be a direct link to him smoking. If you are constantly around a smoker and in intimate settings keep your basis covered by taking NAC (N-Acetyl-L-Cysteine) which provides antioxidant support and vitamin C everyday particularly after kissing. We all should take a regimen after kissing someone ergo who really knows where their mouth has been before yours. ☺

The Sick Headache

I love the TV show Bewitched. One of my favorite lines from the sitcom is when Darren's mother is telling her husband she's getting one of those sick headaches after seeing something actually levitate. Classic! My uncle needed something for his headache one day. I told him to drink water, He did and instantly the headache started to diminish.

If you are taking multiple prescriptions on a daily basis and each one directs you to consume a glass of water, one glass will not do particularly for the whole day. My friends and family are realizing that a lack of water is the main culprit in their headaches. You could also be lacking in B vitamins and or magnesium. Water has an all-access pass even for that sick headache.

SOCK IT TO THEM

Gentleman if you have to wear socks with sandals in summer I have a few suggestions. The first task is to get a pedicure. My first pedicure was like getting a new pair of feet, and each time afterward it felt the same way…. AWESOME! More men should get pedicures not only for themselves but for their significant other. If you can help it, shape up those feet!

Even after having a pedicure and feeling as though you still need to wear socks with sandals, make sure black dress socks are NOT on the list! Colorful polo socks or long colorful soccer socks can be sexy! Much sexier than black dress socks. Show you can be fun with those cartoon zany sox. Stand out from all of the others and show you're formulated with the "Dare Flare!"

"I am not perfect nor do I want to be. The fall from grace is longer with more pieces to pick up"

~Stan D.

DANCE FOR THE MEMORIES

The Luther Vandross song entitled "DANCE WITH MY FATHER AGAIN" hits home with me. My mother Mrs. Cecelia Dixon and I danced together at parties and had the best time. This has given me the fondest of memories. This unconventional suggestion may be the hardest for some to do, but not impossible. Get everyone in your family and dance. No video game dancing. From the grandparents to the kids get together and dance to today's and yesterday's music. There is a special healing process with dancing for all ages. I learned not to judge or laugh at others if their dancing seems odd, it brings a smile to my face to know they are healing. If you are a good dancer, share your energy with others and they will be thankful for the memories.

FORGIVENESS

When we have been wronged by someone we have every right in the world to feel anger towards them. Yes, for what they've done we can preach the schematics of what is right and what is wrong. It feels good to be in power and to reprimand. The key is to forgive that person immediately especially if you're planning to talk, see or be seen with that person in the future. Instantly forgive that person if possible. Each situation is different but try not to prolong a grudge ergo it off-sets your wellbeing as well as with others in your life. There are psychosomatic illnesses caused by unresolved conflicts in life. They are real, not imaginary. Wouldn't you want someone to forgive you for something stupid you've done? ☺

Glutamine, You're Right On Time

Glutamine is one of the few nutrients that can get pass the blood brain barrier. It is food for the brain. Before any surgery I suggest to friends to stop taking their supplements except maybe their multivitamin. To be really certain ask your doctor what is the pre-surgery protocol.

Once your surgery is successful, immediately ask your physician's permission to add Glutamine to your road to recovery. It is a great wound healer along with vitamin C. Glutamine helps with fibroblast (new cells that help produce fibers). The results of my experience with Glutamine has been less muscle wasting. I did not crave any sweets. Unknowingly, I avoided them, I'm talking <u>no cravings</u>. Remember always ask your doctor before starting any new supplement.

GOT NIPPLES?

This is the spiciest I'm going to get in this volume. It lightly touches upon the subject of nipples, - pun was intended. Man or woman if your nipples are sensitive in a good sensual way you have been giving a gift! My nipples were never sensitive until one day someone worked them until I saw the star Orion and Jane Fonda in her Barberella costume flashing before my eyes! It was amazing.

Not to go too much into detail, but the transition was slow and gentle, not rushed and rough. Although some people like it that way, I wouldn't suggest starting out that way. I used warm water or saliva, 2 small nipple suction cups called "snake bites" (anywhere camping gear or adult toys are sold) they don't hurt at all. Lube the rim of the "snake bite" with saliva or warm water then lightly squeezed the "snake bite" on to each nipple. I was not sure so I suctioned them on and off every couple of minutes. My nipples became very sensitive, and things seemed so much more erotic. You can do this yourself or with someone else. Make a play date out of it!☺

HEAD AND SHOULDERS-
OH MY!

If you start using collagen products over time you may have carte blanche to use a light scrub on your face and body, ergo collagen gives your skin the materials for repair. It's like glue for your body. I noticed my skin has a shorter bounce back time from everyday damage from chlorine, sweating, shaving because of supplementation of collagen.

One day I ran out of body wash so I had to use Head and Shoulders. On my wash cloth I squirted a little H&S, brown sugar and lemon juice (natural lemon juice unadulterated without preservatives or a whole lemon will always do.) Before applying the regimen, I wet my hair and body to open pores, than turn the shower off and proceed with a slow light circular motion over my entire body. That's a perfect time to shave for men or women. It will however sting somewhat, but that's the lemon brightening up your skin, and the H&S will start the road to healthy skin because of the main ingredient pyrithione. I have not found pyrithione in the stores yet, but have seen it on line. So for now, I use Head & Shoulders or any brand that contains pyrithione. A dermatologist gave me kudos for using head and shoulders as a body wash. If it's good for the scalp, why not the whole body? ☺

HEART TO HEART

Over the years as a health enthusiast I have come to realize we sometimes can be looked upon as therapist. I just give a listening ear without bias comments or diagnosing. Its not in my scope of practice.   Now I have the chance to give a general overview of what I always wanted to say to women dealing with friends, family and work issues. I can recall a conversation with a woman who said she thinks women were put on this earth to bear children raise them, wither and die.   WOW!   I don't think that way, but from friends, family and the consistency of television it seems to promote that idea.

My mother did not and would not do everything for me. She taught me how to be resourceful. When you incorporate being self-sufficient in your family values you don't get lost in your family. It helps you and them. My mother still did whatever made her happy and still was a great mother. She let everyone know including my dad that we needed to meet her half way. Women are multi-talented but you don't want to get to the point where you hit that "Bitch of a bearing wall" MOMMIE DEAREST. Invest in yourself and not just with shoes or clothes but with mammograms and pap smears.

When you have a doctor's appointment make a freaking day out of it if you can. Go to a spa or movie afterwards. Remember there are herbs placed on earth that are here to help women. From my heart to your heart take more magnesium citrate! (FOR HEART HEALTH) Take advantage of what's accessible to you. RESEARCH!

ALWAYS check with your doctor before trying any new supplements!

LADYS AND GENTS

GLUTATHIONE!

Ladies and gentleman may I introduce Glutathione! It is the amino acid that could have a direct mortality rate among Cancer, HIV and other life - threatening diseases. I'm going into my story telling like Sophia of the "Golden Girls" Picture it …..Springfield Virginia 2008. A group of tourist from Japan came into the health food store that I managed buying up glutathione. It is too costly In Japan. One of the gentleman was very fluent in English, and he explained that the price of glutathione is triple in Japan.

In Japan they are finding how much Glutathione impacts health. At around thirty five dollars a bottle U.S. currency that's a lot of money that many of us do not have. So I did a little research and found out that NAC a much more economical amino acid actually turns into glutathione in your body almost like when beta carotene turns into vitamin A when your body needs it. I read somewhere the transition may work better in men than in women. AS WITH ANY NEW REGIMINE CONSULT A KNOWLEDGABLE

PHYSICIAN BEFORE TRYING!

JAZZING UP THE UNJAZZABLE

FROZEN PIZZZA

I always frowned upon frozen pizza particularly since I live in Philadelphia, home of pizza and cheese-steaks. I did a taste test on the cheapest frozen pizza I could find, - a ninety nine cent pizza to be exact. My father helped me with the taste test. It was a pepperoni pizza that was for a conventional or microwave oven. I followed the directions exactly. I waited with baited breath until it was done. The moment of truth arrived. I took a bite, and it was <u>bland Ville</u>.

I made another attempt and retrieved another pizza from the freezer. I unpackaged it, but this time I rolled butter on the bottom crust, lightly covering it. I also lightly sprinkled garlic powder on the bottom crust. I then flipped the pizza back with the topping side up. I followed the same cooking directions and, WOW a totally different pizza! The crust was the best part. It was flavorful and crisp. My father really tore into it, and he <u>is</u> <u>not</u> a pizza guy especially frozen pizza.

No lame` during the day

Madame, you are infringing on my constitutional rights by wearing lame` and other such apparel during daytime hours. It is heart wrenching and disturbing to see that some women do not know not to wear shiny clothing during the day, especially on sunny days. Please, please, please save all shiny couture for the evening so you can brightening up the night life with your radiant inner and outer beauty. Remember no more than two items of your outfit should shine, so do not overkill!

"As cute as I am…. Don't let me have to get ugly"☺

~Stan D.

Taking supplements before bed

I'm a firm believer in taking supplements before bed. It is a critical time of day to assist with the body's healing process. My friends and family are my personal clinical trials but don't tell them it's our secret. My kin always say they wake up super earlier than usual and don't need their alarm clock to up root them from their slumber. My family members realize that they are supplying the body with materials for recovery.

Incorporate a regimen that consists of amino acids, antioxidants and vitamin D. These items repair, rejuvenate and reload. You may not get immediate gratification but from my experience, who, ever did a night regimen benefited in some way or another. I'm usually a capsule man I break open the capsule in a protein shake, fruit drink or a nighttime tea (Luke warm) for a faster dispersal. The amino acid complex will help with muscle and tissue rebuilding especially benefiting the skin. The antioxidants will quench the free radicals of your day. I would add about 500 to 1000 mg of vitamin C, because it is used for so many things in the body so you will want to have enough to go around. It helps the Immune system and repairing of skin just to name a few. I know of people supplementing up to six thousand mg a day- but for now I would suggest 500 to 1000mg. Five years ago I realized that vitamin D was important when a doctor came into the health store that I managed and almost bought our entire line of vitamin D for his family. He explained that a deficiency of vitamin D is being studied as the leading cause of an array of diseases that we are still encountering today. Remember folks, this was five years ago! WOW. Ask a physician that's knowledgeable in supplements.☺

ADDED SUPPLEMENTS

1. GINSENG
2. GLUTAMINE

TAXING MY BRAIN

If you are receiving unemployment compensation, make certain you are getting taxes deducted. Many people are receiving an unemployment check and not realizing taxes are not being subtracted. There should be in your profile the amount you would like taken out. I understand you need to maximize as much as possible from your unemployment checks, but it will be in your best interest to get those federal and state taxes taken out. I even brought it to the attention of a new IRS worker who said when she goes on furlough and receives unemployment that she should have taxes taken out. ☺

THE SKINNY ON MEDICATION

Anyone in the medical field knows research done on multiple medications that you may take is nonexistent except maybe if the meds are to work in synergist with one another. First, I would like to say, Love your doctor. They are human, compassionate and busy! You are not the only patient on their plate. When you are prescribed meds, it is up to you to research them and find out the pros and cons and testimonies of others who may have used encountered the same medication. Most medications are prescribed to be taking for a limited time, with periodic evaluation.

I was dining in a restaurant and overheard a conversation after a gentleman ordered his cholesterol- filled meal. He was boasting about why he's not worried about his cholesterol levels he's taking a <u>statin</u> drug. That tells me he is willingly dependent on that pill for cholesterol control. Statin drugs may inhibit cholesterol production in the liver but it may also inhibit Coenzyme Q10 production (antioxidant) as well which is also produced in the liver and vital for heart function.

On Each doctors visit ask him or her what meds can you omit. Also ask yourself where do your meds go after taking them? Some reappear in that pouch area near the stomach in the lower abdominal region.   DETOX! DETOX! DETOX! Did I mention detox? Get that lymphatic system going helping to get rid of toxins and medication byproducts? The results can be great health, weight loss and other perks that comes different with each individual.

THE WHAT TO DO!

These are a few suggestions of what to do before going to the doctor. Omit coffee or products that contain caffeine! Omit sodas or anything containing sugar except for suggestions at the end of this excerpt. From accompanying my father and uncle on doctor's appointments, I observed that the doctor only knows what you tell them and their tests do not lie! Picture a scenario of you having a cup of coffee or two before seeing the doctor. You had to rush a little to make that appointment. Adrenal glands kick in and your anxiety levels just hit the wall. When they take your blood- pressure- reading, it <u>may</u> <u>be</u> elevated. As you may already know anything other than 120 over 60 or 110 over 80 will put your doctor in concern mode.   Always get to your doctor's appointment early than your scheduled time so that you can relax and be ahead of the game. Sometimes without you even knowing, Iatrophobia…. the fear of doctors, can set in and your vitals can be off the chart!

If you are getting a glucose test any added sugar could spike your glucose reading. Insulin reading above seven could land you on medication and all you may have had was a glass of orange juice.

I'm suggesting this for people whose blood pressure and insulin readings are already normal. Before your appointment Water and wheat cereal (naturally lightly sweetened with no more than 5grams of sugar per serving). If you have a special diet that the doctor placed you on follow your doctor's suggestions. Good luck. ALWAYS CONSULT YOUR DOCTOR BEFORE TRYING ANY SUGGESTIONS. ☺

THE UNCONVENTIONAL BREAKFAST

No matter what I eat for breakfast, I started incorporating a small salad that consists of kale, onion and shredded carrots. Not only am I increasing my fiber intake, but I'm also feeding and rejuvenating my enzymes and probiotics with raw veggies. If I keep this daily regimen my body is sure to go thru a metamorphosis. If I have eggs and bacon, I'm going to have my salad. If I have just a protein shake for breakfast, I will have my house salad with it.

It started making sense to me to eat more foods that are alive i.e. vegetables to justify the cooked foods I ate. Vegetables are connected with nutrient co-factors that are vital to our wellbeing and mortality rate. What we eat for breakfast can set the tone for the rest of our day. ☺

YOU CAN'T SHAKE THIS

People look like this ☹ when it's time to drink their protein shake. So let's try and remedy that by simply adding green tea ginger ale (I used a vanilla shake). It's probably the only soda my dad and I drink. It tastes crisp and natural and it contains 200 mg of antioxidants. WOW! When I add this to our protein shake it drastically changes the taste. It's almost like drinking a root beer float but lighter and healthier. My father finishes it in no time flat. I start out with a blender containing the directed amount of protein with milk for two people. I add two alive men's multi vitamin and two squirts of chloroxygen to help with dispersement of the protein (not needed if you don't have it). Blend and add protein and soda to desired taste. The ginger ale helps digestion of the protein and the green tea helps with the antioxidants side of things. The point is to add things to your shake for a great taste and nutrient enhancement. ☺

NUMBER 2

Oddly enough a cab driver and I got on the subject of what is normal to frequent the bathroom primarily to do "number 2". After witnessing an overweight teen walking in front of the cab, the cab driver and I were in agreement that the teen looked to be unhealthy. That was our Segway onto the topics of health and fitness. Then onto the topic of frequenting the bathroom. I personally think you should go to the bathroom the same amount of times you eat in a day. That depends on whether you have an adequate water and fiber intake or if your digestive enzymes are in full swing.

Fortunately when I consume a meal number 2 is not far behind...... pun <u>was</u> intended. I feel much better and non-lethargic when having a complete healthy bowel movement. Loose or acorn shaped bowel movements are a sign of poor digestion.
For some it's all too easy but for others it's an uphill battle. Train your body to eliminate frequently and efficiently. <u>Ask a Physician what is the protocol for elimination.</u>

<u>WEAPONS OF CHOICE</u>

1. 64 ounces of water a day
2. Fiber and digestive enzymes taken with each meal.

"I am alkaline. Cancer cannot live in me!"

~Stan D.

INNOCUOS INFO!

1. Once a year get your vitamin and mineral levels checked.

2. Your diet is your life style you do not go on and off it. As long as you're consuming something you're always on a diet. Tell people you're going on a detox to get healthier and to lose weight. Then they will know you're serious about the subject.

3. Ladies and Gents, when you have an event approaching check your shoe-wear days prior. You may have to get your shoes professionally shined or de-scuffed.   A Scuffed or worn shoe blows the whole outfit!   Remember you can wear a paper bag but with a hot unscuffed shoe you're the sexiest in the room.

4. If you or loved one is sick, albeit a common cold to a chronic illness make sure you have air circulating in the room. Stagnant bacteria fills the air. Place a small fan on the floor so air would not blow directly on the person who has

taking ill. Only use white sheets and pillowcases. Change linen every morning without fail. Do not use laundry detergent to wash only bleach and hot water. Fresh white cotton linen is therapeutic.

5. Punk -ish -ment
    (Plural punkishments)

A. The penalty adult friends give to one another if someone has done adolescent wrong doings. *i.e. Not showing up for birthdays, forgetting anniversaries, never calling to say hello. In other words, **F**king up!***

B. You first forgive the individual, then give them a calendar day when they are allowed to communicate with you again. If you stick to the calendar day that was given they will think twice about being irresponsible towards you again!

THANK YOU!

GOD!
Cecelia Dixon
Wilbert Webb
Carl Dixon Sr.
Carl Dixon Jr.
Sondra Dixon
My beautiful sister in-law "SANDY"
My nieces and nephews
Jaime Campbell (your so matter of fact)
All the staff at Mazzonni
Dr. Caroline (You are an angel. I see your wings whenever
I see you!)
Dr. Goodman
Dr. Dusty Lattimmer (Thank You!!)
My cousins…Bobby, Charlotte, Deare, Leslee and Theresa
(You guys in your own way, kept me going!)
Aunt Frances
Dr. William Short
Mr. Jeffrey "freshness" Deitrich (Thanks for the love and
support in bringing this to fruition.)
My family at the Woods Campground
James "Sonny" Peel
Jeff Anders
Last and certainly not least Mr. Michael Ceretelli (A true
friend even thru the stupid mistakes I've made)
Tasha

References

ROBERT GRAY
THE COLON HANDBOOK
(TWELFTH REVISED EDITION)
EMERALD PUBLISHING
RENO NEVADA

Mommy Dearest
Paramount pictures

Golden Girls
NBC, Lifetime